THE COPD

DIET

COOKBOOK

SARAH JACK

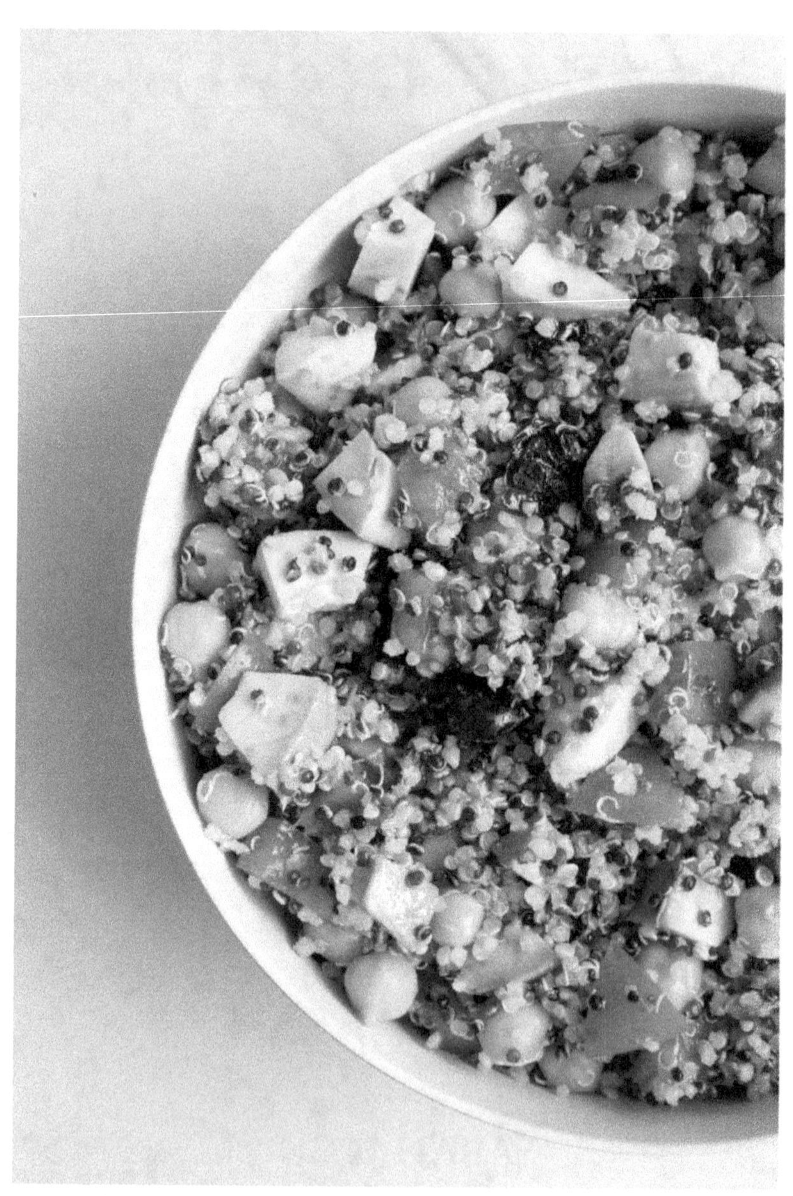

COPYRIGHT

3

All rights reserved. This book or any portion thereof may

not be reproduced or used in any manner whatsoever

without the express written permission of the publisher

except for the use of brief quotations in a book review.

TABLE OF CONTENTS

Table of Contents

INTRODUCTION

LUNGS

The lungs are crucial organs within the respiratory system responsible for facilitating the exchange of oxygen and carbon dioxide between the air we inhale and our bloodstream. Here are some key aspects regarding the lungs:

Anatomy: Situated in the chest cavity on either side of the heart, the lungs are spongy, cone-shaped structures. Each lung is segmented into lobes – three on the right (upper, middle, and lower) and two on the left (upper and lower).

Function: The primary role of the lungs is to enable the exchange of gases during breathing. As air is drawn in, it travels through the trachea, bronchi, and bronchioles until reaching tiny air sacs called alveoli. Oxygen crosses the thin alveolar walls into the bloodstream, while carbon dioxide, a metabolic byproduct, moves from the bloodstream into the alveoli to be exhaled.

Respiratory System: Comprising the airways (trachea, bronchi, and bronchioles), diaphragm, and other respiratory muscles, the lungs are integral to the broader respiratory system. Together, these components facilitate oxygen intake and carbon dioxide removal.

Protection and Defense: Various mechanisms safeguard the lungs from harmful substances. The mucous lining traps particles and pathogens, while cilia help to sweep debris from the airways. Immune cells within the lungs identify and neutralize invading pathogens.

Respiratory Disorders: Numerous diseases and conditions can affect lung health, including infections (pneumonia, tuberculosis), chronic lung ailments (COPD, asthma, bronchitis), lung cancer, pulmonary embolism, and respiratory distress syndrome. Factors like smoking, air pollution, occupational hazards, and genetic predispositions contribute to these disorders.

In summary, the lungs are pivotal for maintaining oxygen levels, expelling carbon dioxide, and supporting overall health. Protecting lung health through measures such as avoiding smoking, minimizing exposure to pollutants, and promptly addressing respiratory issues is crucial for optimal well-being.

COPD

COPD, or Chronic Obstructive Pulmonary Disease, is a chronic respiratory condition characterized by persistent airflow obstruction in the lungs, which typically worsens over time and is not completely reversible. This disease primarily comprises two main conditions: chronic bronchitis and emphysema.

Chronic Bronchitis: Chronic bronchitis involves long-standing inflammation and irritation of the bronchial tubes, the air passages that carry air to and from the lungs. This inflammation leads to increased production of mucus, which can block the airways and result in symptoms such as coughing and difficulty breathing.

Emphysema: Emphysema, on the other hand, entails damage to the air sacs (alveoli) in the lungs. Prolonged exposure to irritants like cigarette smoke or environmental pollutants can cause these air sacs to lose their elasticity, impairing the lungs' ability to expand and contract effectively. This damage results in decreased airflow and compromised gas exchange, leading to symptoms like shortness of breath and wheezing.

Common symptoms of COPD include persistent cough, shortness of breath (particularly during physical exertion), wheezing, chest tightness, and susceptibility to respiratory infections.

COPD is primarily caused by prolonged exposure to irritants such as cigarette smoke, secondhand smoke, air pollution, and occupational hazards like dust and chemicals. Genetic factors may also contribute to an individual's susceptibility to developing COPD.

Diagnosis of COPD typically involves a comprehensive assessment, including medical history evaluation, physical examination, lung function tests (such as spirometry), and imaging studies (such as chest X-rays or CT scans).

Treatment for COPD focuses on alleviating symptoms, enhancing quality of life, and slowing disease progression. Strategies may include:

Smoking Cessation: Quitting smoking is paramount in managing COPD and preventing further lung damage.

Medications: Bronchodilators and inhaled corticosteroids help relax and open the airways, reducing inflammation in the lungs.

Pulmonary Rehabilitation: Structured programs involving exercise, education, and support can enhance respiratory function and overall physical fitness.

Oxygen Therapy: Supplemental oxygen may be necessary in advanced cases to improve blood oxygen levels.

Surgical Interventions: Lung volume reduction surgery or lung transplantation may be considered for select individuals with severe COPD.

Early diagnosis and intervention are crucial in managing COPD effectively and improving outcomes. Individuals experiencing symptoms suggestive of COPD should seek prompt medical evaluation and treatment to optimize their lung health and overall well-being.

COPD DIET

A dietary regimen for COPD (Chronic Obstructive Pulmonary Disease) is centered around providing appropriate nutrition to bolster overall well-being and address symptoms linked to the condition. Here are some dietary guidelines for individuals managing COPD:

Nutrient-Rich Diet: Embrace a well-rounded diet featuring ample servings of fruits, vegetables, whole grains, lean proteins, and healthy fats. This dietary approach ensures the intake of essential nutrients like vitamins, minerals, antioxidants, and fiber, which are vital for supporting overall health and bolstering the immune system.

Healthy Fats: Integrate sources of beneficial fats such as avocados, nuts, seeds, olive oil, and fatty fish like salmon or trout. These fats possess anti-inflammatory properties and supply crucial fatty acids that promote lung health.

Protein-Rich Foods: Incorporate protein-rich foods such as poultry, fish, eggs, legumes, tofu, and dairy products into your meals. Protein aids in maintaining muscle strength and tissue repair, which can be particularly beneficial for individuals experiencing muscle weakness or weight loss due to COPD.

Hydration: Ensure adequate hydration by consuming plenty of fluids throughout the day, with a preference for water. Proper hydration assists in thinning mucus secretions, facilitating easier breathing, and reducing the likelihood of exacerbations.

Small, Frequent Meals: Opt for smaller, more frequent meals over large ones to mitigate bloating and discomfort, factors that can exacerbate breathing difficulties in individuals with COPD.

Sodium Moderation: Monitor and limit sodium intake, as excess sodium can contribute to fluid retention and exacerbate symptoms such as shortness of breath. Focus on minimizing processed foods, canned soups, and high-sodium condiments in favor of fresh, whole food options.

Weight Management: Strive to maintain a healthy weight to alleviate strain on the respiratory system. Depending on your weight status, work towards increasing calorie and nutrient intake with nutrient-dense foods if underweight, or collaborate with healthcare providers to establish a gradual, sustainable weight loss plan if overweight.

Avoidance of Gas-Producing Foods: Some individuals with COPD may experience discomfort and bloating from gas-producing foods like beans, cabbage, broccoli, and carbonated beverages. Monitor your symptoms and limit intake of these foods if they exacerbate your condition.

Vitamin D: Ensure adequate levels of vitamin D, crucial for lung health and immune function. Incorporate foods rich in vitamin D such as fatty fish, egg yolks, fortified dairy products, and expose yourself to sunlight, or discuss vitamin D supplementation with your healthcare provider if needed.

Consultation with a Registered Dietitian: Seek personalized dietary guidance tailored to your specific health needs and circumstances by consulting with a registered dietitian. They can develop a comprehensive nutrition plan to support your COPD management, in collaboration with your healthcare team comprising your primary care physician, pulmonologist, and other specialists.

It's paramount to collaborate closely with healthcare professionals to devise a COPD diet strategy that caters to your individual nutritional requirements and contributes to optimizing your overall health and well-being.

BENEFITS OF COPD DIET

The benefits of adhering to a COPD diet tailored to meet the specific requirements of individuals with Chronic Obstructive Pulmonary Disease (COPD) encompass:

Nutritional Support: A COPD diet furnishes vital nutrients crucial for overall health, including essential vitamins, minerals, antioxidants, and protein. This nutritional support bolsters immune function, facilitates tissue repair, and preserves muscle strength, which holds significance for COPD patients.

Weight Management: A well-rounded COPD diet aids individuals in attaining and sustaining a healthy weight. It assists underweight individuals in augmenting calorie intake to avert malnutrition and muscle depletion. Conversely, for overweight individuals, the diet facilitates gradual weight reduction to alleviate strain on the respiratory system.

Optimized Lung Function: Certain nutrients like omega-3 fatty acids from fatty fish and antioxidants sourced from fruits and vegetables possess anti-inflammatory attributes that might mitigate lung inflammation and enhance respiratory function among COPD patients.

Improved Respiratory Symptoms: Adherence to a COPD diet incorporating lung-supportive foods such as fruits, vegetables, whole grains, and lean proteins may help alleviate respiratory symptoms like breathlessness and coughing commonly associated with COPD.

Enhanced Hydration: Adequate hydration, underscored by a COPD diet, plays a pivotal role in thinning mucus secretions within the airways, facilitating easier breathing, and diminishing the likelihood of exacerbations. The diet emphasizes maintaining optimal hydration levels by consuming ample fluids throughout the day.

Reduced Risk of Complications: By steering clear of foods that exacerbate symptoms, such as high-sodium items or gas-inducing foods, COPD individuals can mitigate the risk of complications like fluid retention, bloating, and discomfort.

Enhanced Quality of Life: Adhering to a personalized COPD diet tailored to individual preferences and needs can enhance quality of life by furnishing the energy and nutrients requisite for daily activities, alleviating symptoms impeding daily functioning, and fostering overall well-being.

Long-Term Health Management: Integrating healthy dietary practices into COPD management confers enduring benefits for overall health, potentially diminishing the likelihood of complications and disease progression associated with COPD.

It's imperative for COPD patients to collaborate closely with their healthcare team, including a registered dietitian, to devise a customized COPD diet plan aligning with their unique nutritional needs and health objectives. Regular monitoring and adjustments to the diet may be necessary contingent upon alterations in symptoms, medication regimens, and overall health status.

EXERCISE AND LUNG HEALTH

Physical activity and exercise play a crucial role in maintaining lung health and function. Here are some key points highlighting the relationship between exercise and lung health:

Improved Lung Function: Regular exercise can enhance lung capacity and efficiency by strengthening the respiratory muscles and increasing the volume of air the lungs can hold. This leads to improved oxygen exchange and better overall lung function.

Reduced Risk of Respiratory Conditions: Engaging in regular physical activity has been shown to reduce the risk of developing respiratory conditions such as chronic obstructive pulmonary disease (COPD), asthma, and bronchitis. Exercise helps to keep the airways clear, improves circulation, and strengthens the immune system, reducing susceptibility to respiratory infections.

Enhanced Respiratory Muscle Strength: Exercise, particularly aerobic and resistance training, strengthens the muscles involved in breathing, such as the diaphragm and intercostal muscles. Stronger respiratory muscles require less effort to breathe, reducing fatigue and shortness of breath during physical activity and daily tasks.

Improved Exercise Tolerance: Regular exercise improves cardiovascular fitness and endurance, allowing individuals to engage in physical activities for longer durations without experiencing breathlessness or fatigue. This increased exercise tolerance can lead to a more active lifestyle and better overall health.

Better Management of Existing Lung Conditions: For individuals with existing lung conditions such as COPD or asthma, exercise is an essential component of pulmonary rehabilitation programs. These programs typically include a combination of aerobic exercise, strength training, and breathing exercises designed to improve symptoms, enhance quality of life, and reduce the frequency of exacerbations.

Promotion of Lung Health Across the Lifespan: Regular physical activity from childhood through adulthood can help maintain optimal lung health and function as individuals age. Encouraging children and adolescents to engage in regular physical activity can establish healthy habits that carry into adulthood, reducing the risk of respiratory problems later in life.

Support for Smoking Cessation: Exercise can aid in smoking cessation efforts by reducing nicotine cravings and withdrawal symptoms. Engaging in physical activity provides a healthy alternative to smoking and can help individuals manage stress and anxiety associated with quitting smoking.

Overall Health Benefits: In addition to its direct impact on lung health, exercise offers numerous other health benefits, including weight management, improved cardiovascular health, reduced risk of chronic diseases such as diabetes and hypertension, and enhanced mental well-being.

In conclusion, regular exercise is essential for maintaining lung health, improving respiratory function, and reducing the risk of respiratory conditions. Incorporating a variety of physical activities into one's routine, along with adopting a healthy lifestyle, can contribute to optimal lung health and overall well-being.

COPD DIET RECIPES

Quinoa Salad with Avocado and Chickpeas

Ingredients:

- 1 cup quinoa, rinsed

- 1 can chickpeas, drained and rinsed

- 1 ripe avocado, diced

- 1/2 cup cherry tomatoes, halved

- 1/4 cup chopped fresh cilantro

- 2 tablespoons olive oil

- 1 tablespoon lemon juice

- Salt and pepper to taste

Instructions:

- Cook quinoa according to package instructions and let it cool.

- In a large bowl, combine quinoa, chickpeas, avocado, cherry tomatoes, and cilantro.

- In a small bowl, whisk together olive oil, lemon juice, salt, and pepper.

- Pour the dressing over the quinoa salad and toss gently to combine. Serve chilled.

Baked Salmon with Asparagus

Ingredients:

- 4 salmon fillets

- 1 bunch asparagus, trimmed

- 2 tablespoons olive oil

- 2 cloves garlic, minced

- 1 teaspoon lemon zest

- Salt and pepper to taste

Instructions:

- Preheat the oven to 400°F (200°C).

- Place the salmon fillets and asparagus on a baking sheet.

- In a small bowl, mix together olive oil, minced garlic, lemon zest, salt, and pepper.

- Brush the olive oil mixture over the salmon and asparagus.

- Bake for 12-15 minutes or until the salmon is cooked through and the asparagus is tender. Serve hot.

Vegetable Stir-Fry with Tofu

Ingredients:

- 1 block firm tofu, cubed

- 2 cups mixed vegetables (such as bell peppers, broccoli, carrots)

- 2 tablespoons soy sauce

- 1 tablespoon sesame oil

- 2 cloves garlic, minced

- 1 teaspoon grated ginger

- Cooked brown rice for serving

Instructions:

- Heat sesame oil in a large skillet over medium heat.

- Add tofu cubes and cook until golden brown on all sides.

Remove tofu from the skillet and set aside.

- In the same skillet, add a bit more sesame oil if needed, then add minced garlic and grated ginger. Cook for 1 minute.

- Add mixed vegetables to the skillet and stir-fry until tender.

- Return the cooked tofu to the skillet and add soy sauce. Stir to combine.

- Serve the vegetable stir-fry over cooked brown rice.

Chicken and Vegetable Soup

Ingredients:

- 2 chicken breasts, cooked and shredded

- 4 cups chicken broth

- 1 onion, diced

- 2 carrots, sliced

- 2 celery stalks, sliced

- 1 cup green beans, chopped

- 2 cloves garlic, minced

- 1 teaspoon dried thyme

- Salt and pepper to taste

Instructions:

- In a large pot, heat olive oil over medium heat. Add diced onion, sliced carrots, celery, and minced garlic. Cook until vegetables are softened.

- Add shredded chicken, chicken broth, dried thyme, salt, and pepper to the pot. Bring to a boil.

- Reduce heat and let the soup simmer for 20-25 minutes.

- Add chopped green beans and continue to simmer for another 10 minutes or until all vegetables are tender.

- Adjust seasoning if needed and serve hot.

Mango and Spinach Smoothie

Ingredients:

- 1 ripe mango, peeled and diced

- 1 cup fresh spinach leaves

- 1/2 cup plain Greek yogurt

- 1/2 cup almond milk

- 1 tablespoon honey (optional)

Instructions:

- Place all ingredients in a blender.

- Blend until smooth and creamy.

- Taste and add honey if additional sweetness is desired.

- Pour into glasses and serve immediately.

Cauliflower and Broccoli Crust Pizza

Ingredients:

- 1 small head cauliflower, grated

- 1 small head broccoli, grated

- 2 eggs

- 1/2 cup shredded cheese (such as mozzarella)

- 1 teaspoon dried Italian herbs

- Pizza sauce, cheese, and toppings of your choice

Instructions:

- Preheat oven to 400°F (200°C). Line a baking sheet with parchment paper.

- In a large bowl, mix together grated cauliflower, grated broccoli, eggs, shredded cheese, and dried Italian herbs until well combined.

- Spread the cauliflower and broccoli mixture onto the prepared baking sheet, shaping it into a round crust.

- Bake the crust for 25-30 minutes or until golden brown and firm.

- Remove from the oven and top with pizza sauce, cheese, and your favorite toppings.

- Return to the oven and bake for an additional 10-15 minutes or until the cheese is melted and bubbly.

- Slice and serve cauliflower and broccoli crust pizza hot.

Turmeric Chicken with Roasted Vegetables

Ingredients:

- 4 boneless, skinless chicken breasts

- 2 tablespoons olive oil

- 1 tablespoon turmeric powder

- 1 teaspoon paprika

- 1 teaspoon ground cumin

- 1 teaspoon garlic powder

- 1 teaspoon onion powder

- Salt and pepper to taste

- 4 cups mixed vegetables (such as carrots, Brussels sprouts, and cauliflower), chopped

Instructions:

- Preheat oven to 400°F (200°C). Line a baking sheet with parchment paper.

- In a small bowl, mix together olive oil, turmeric powder, paprika, ground cumin, garlic powder, onion powder, salt, and pepper.

- Place chicken breasts on one side of the prepared baking sheet and coat them with the turmeric spice mixture.

- On the other side of the baking sheet, spread chopped mixed vegetables and drizzle with olive oil. Season with salt and pepper.

- Roast in the oven for 25-30 minutes or until the chicken is cooked through and the vegetables are tender.

- Serve turmeric chicken with roasted vegetables hot.

Eggplant and Tomato Casserole

Ingredients:

- 2 large eggplants, sliced

- 2 tomatoes, sliced

- 1 onion, thinly sliced

- 2 cloves garlic, minced

- 1/2 cup breadcrumbs

- 1/4 cup grated Parmesan cheese

- 2 tablespoons olive oil

- 1 teaspoon dried oregano

- Salt and pepper to taste

Instructions:

- Preheat oven to 375°F (190°C). Grease a baking dish with olive oil.

- Arrange sliced eggplants in the bottom of the baking dish, overlapping slightly.

- Layer sliced tomatoes on top of the eggplants, followed by thinly sliced onions and minced garlic.

- In a small bowl, mix together breadcrumbs, grated Parmesan cheese, dried oregano, salt, and pepper.

- Sprinkle the breadcrumb mixture over the top of the vegetables.

- Drizzle olive oil over the breadcrumb topping.

- Cover the baking dish with foil and bake for 30 minutes.

- Remove foil and bake for an additional 15-20 minutes or until the top is golden brown and the vegetables are tender.

- Serve eggplant and tomato casserole hot.

Miso Glazed Salmon with Steamed Vegetables

Ingredients:

- 4 salmon fillets

- 2 tablespoons miso paste

- 2 tablespoons soy sauce

- 1 tablespoon honey

- 1 tablespoon rice vinegar

- 2 cloves garlic, minced

- 1 teaspoon grated ginger

- Steamed vegetables of your choice (such as broccoli, carrots, and snow peas)

Instructions:

- Preheat the oven to 400°F (200°C).

- In a small bowl, whisk together miso paste, soy sauce, honey, rice vinegar, minced garlic, and grated ginger to make the glaze.

- Place salmon fillets on a baking sheet lined with parchment paper.

- Brush the miso glaze over the salmon fillets.

- Bake for 12-15 minutes or until the salmon is cooked through and flakes easily with a fork.

- Serve the miso glazed salmon with steamed vegetables.

Sesame Ginger Beef Stir-Fry

Ingredients:

- 1 lb beef sirloin, thinly sliced

- 2 tablespoons soy sauce

- 1 tablespoon sesame oil

- 2 cloves garlic, minced

- 1 tablespoon grated ginger

- 2 cups mixed vegetables (such as bell peppers, snap peas, and mushrooms), sliced

- Cooked brown rice for serving

- Sesame seeds for garnish

Instructions:

- In a bowl, marinate sliced beef sirloin with soy sauce and sesame oil for 15-20 minutes.

- Heat a tablespoon of sesame oil in a large skillet or wok over high heat.

- Add minced garlic and grated ginger to the skillet and cook for 1 minute.

- Add marinated beef slices to the skillet and stir-fry until browned.

- Add mixed vegetables to the skillet and stir-fry until tender-crisp.

- Serve sesame ginger beef stir-fry over cooked brown rice, garnished with sesame seeds.

Coconut Curry Lentil Soup

Ingredients:

- 1 cup dried red lentils, rinsed

- 1 onion, diced

- 2 carrots, diced

- 2 cloves garlic, minced

- 1 tablespoon curry powder

- 1 teaspoon ground turmeric

- 1 can (14 oz) coconut milk

- 4 cups vegetable broth

- Salt and pepper to taste

- Fresh cilantro for garnish

Instructions:

- In a large pot, heat olive oil over medium heat. Add diced onion, diced carrots, and minced garlic. Cook until softened.

- Add curry powder and ground turmeric to the pot. Stir to combine.

- Add rinsed red lentils, coconut milk, and vegetable broth to the pot. Bring to a boil.

- Reduce heat and let the soup simmer for 20-25 minutes or until the lentils are cooked through.

- Season with salt and pepper to taste.

- Serve coconut curry lentil soup hot, garnished with fresh cilantro.

Baked Cod with Lemon and Herbs

Ingredients:

- 4 cod fillets

- 2 tablespoons olive oil

- 2 tablespoons lemon juice

- 2 cloves garlic, minced

- 1 teaspoon dried thyme

- 1 teaspoon dried oregano

- Salt and pepper to taste

- Lemon slices for garnish

Instructions:

- Preheat the oven to 400°F (200°C).

- In a small bowl, whisk together olive oil, lemon juice, minced garlic, dried thyme, dried oregano, salt, and pepper.

- Place cod fillets on a baking sheet lined with parchment paper.

- Brush the olive oil mixture over the cod fillets.

- Bake for 12-15 minutes or until the cod is cooked through and flakes easily with a fork.

- Serve baked cod with lemon slices.

Tofu and Vegetable Curry

Ingredients:

- 1 block firm tofu, cubed

- 2 cups mixed vegetables (such as bell peppers, broccoli, and cauliflower), chopped

- 1 onion, diced

- 2 cloves garlic, minced

- 1 tablespoon curry powder

- 1 can (14 oz) coconut milk

- 2 tablespoons soy sauce

- 1 tablespoon olive oil

- Cooked rice for serving

- Fresh cilantro for garnish

Instructions:

- In a large skillet, heat olive oil over medium heat. Add diced onion and minced garlic. Cook until softened.

- Add cubed tofu to the skillet and cook until golden brown on all sides.

- Stir in curry powder and cook for 1 minute.

- Add mixed vegetables to the skillet and stir to combine.

- Pour coconut milk and soy sauce over the tofu and vegetables. Bring to a simmer.

- Let the curry simmer for 10-15 minutes or until the vegetables are tender.

- Serve tofu and vegetable curry over cooked rice, garnished with fresh cilantro.

Lemon Garlic Shrimp Pasta

Ingredients:

- 8 oz pasta of your choice

- 1 lb shrimp, peeled and deveined

- 2 tablespoons olive oil

- 4 cloves garlic, minced

- Zest of 1 lemon

- Juice of 1 lemon

- 1/4 cup chopped fresh parsley

- Salt and pepper to taste

Instructions:

- Cook pasta according to package instructions. Drain and set aside.

- In a large skillet, heat olive oil over medium heat. Add minced garlic and cook until fragrant.

- Add shrimp to the skillet and cook until pink and opaque, about 2-3 minutes per side.

- Stir in lemon zest and lemon juice. Season with salt and pepper to taste.

- Add cooked pasta to the skillet and toss to combine.

- Remove from heat and garnish with chopped fresh parsley.

- Serve lemon garlic shrimp pasta hot.

Crispy Baked Eggplant Parmesan

Ingredients:

- 1 large eggplant, sliced into rounds

- 1 cup breadcrumbs

- 1/2 cup grated Parmesan cheese

- 2 eggs, beaten

- 2 cups marinara sauce

- 1 cup shredded mozzarella cheese

- Fresh basil leaves for garnish

Instructions:

- Preheat the oven to 400°F (200°C). Line a baking sheet with parchment paper.

- Dip eggplant slices into beaten eggs, then coat with a mixture of breadcrumbs and grated Parmesan cheese.

- Place coated eggplant slices on the prepared baking sheet and bake for 20-25 minutes or until golden and crispy.

- In a baking dish, spread a layer of marinara sauce. Arrange baked eggplant slices on top of the sauce.

- Spoon more marinara sauce over the eggplant slices and sprinkle with shredded mozzarella cheese.

- Bake for an additional 15-20 minutes or until the cheese is melted and bubbly.

- Garnish with fresh basil leaves before serving.

Chickpea and Vegetable Tagine

Ingredients:

- 1 can (15 oz) chickpeas, drained and rinsed

- 2 carrots, sliced

- 1 onion, diced

- 2 cloves garlic, minced

- 1 tablespoon olive oil

- 1 teaspoon ground cumin

- 1 teaspoon ground coriander

- 1/2 teaspoon ground cinnamon

- 1/4 teaspoon ground turmeric

- 1 can (14 oz) diced tomatoes

- 1 cup vegetable broth

- Salt and pepper to taste

- Cooked couscous for serving

- Fresh cilantro for garnish

Instructions:

- Heat olive oil in a large pot over medium heat. Add diced onion and minced garlic. Cook until softened.

- Add sliced carrots, ground cumin, ground coriander, ground cinnamon, and ground turmeric to the pot. Stir to combine.

- Pour diced tomatoes (with juices) and vegetable broth into the pot. Bring to a simmer.

- Add drained and rinsed chickpeas to the pot. Simmer for 20-25 minutes or until the carrots are tender.

- Season with salt and pepper to taste.

- Serve chickpea and vegetable tagine over cooked couscous, garnished with fresh cilantro.

Creamy Mushroom and Spinach Pasta

Ingredients:

- 8 oz pasta of your choice

- 2 tablespoons butter

- 8 oz mushrooms, sliced

- 2 cloves garlic, minced

- 2 cups fresh spinach

- 1 cup heavy cream

- 1/2 cup grated Parmesan cheese

- Salt and pepper to taste

- Chopped fresh parsley for garnish

Instructions:

- Cook pasta according to package instructions. Drain and set aside.

- In a skillet, melt butter over medium heat. Add sliced mushrooms and minced garlic. Cook until mushrooms are tender.

- Stir in fresh spinach and cook until wilted.

- Pour in heavy cream and grated Parmesan cheese. Stir until the sauce is creamy and heated through.

- Season with salt and pepper to taste.

- Add cooked pasta to the skillet and toss to coat evenly with the sauce.

- Garnish with chopped fresh parsley before serving.

Roasted Butternut Squash and Apple Soup

Ingredients:

- 1 butternut squash, peeled, seeded, and cubed

- 2 apples, peeled, cored, and cubed

- 1 onion, diced

- 2 cloves garlic, minced

- 4 cups vegetable broth

- 1 teaspoon ground cinnamon

- 1/2 teaspoon ground nutmeg

- Salt and pepper to taste

- Olive oil for roasting

- Greek yogurt for garnish (optional)

Instructions:

- Preheat the oven to 400°F (200°C).

- Place cubed butternut squash, cubed apples, and diced onion on a baking sheet.

- Drizzle with olive oil and toss to coat evenly. Season with salt and pepper.

- Roast in the oven for 25-30 minutes or until the vegetables are tender and caramelized.

- Transfer roasted vegetables to a large pot. Add minced garlic, vegetable broth, ground cinnamon, and ground nutmeg.

- Bring to a simmer and cook for 10-15 minutes.

- Use an immersion blender to puree the soup until smooth. Alternatively, transfer the soup in batches to a blender and puree until smooth.

- Season with additional salt and pepper if needed.

- Serve roasted butternut squash and apple soup hot, garnished with a dollop of Greek yogurt if desired.

Salmon and Quinoa Salad with Lemon Dijon Dressing

Ingredients:

- 2 salmon fillets

- 1 cup quinoa, cooked

- 2 cups mixed greens

- 1 cucumber, diced

- 1/4 cup cherry tomatoes, halved

- 2 tablespoons olive oil

- 1 tablespoon lemon juice

- 1 teaspoon Dijon mustard

- Salt and pepper to taste

Instructions:

- Preheat the oven to 375°F (190°C). Place salmon fillets on a baking sheet, season with salt and pepper, and bake for 12-15 minutes or until cooked through.

- In a large bowl, combine cooked quinoa, mixed greens, diced cucumber, and cherry tomatoes.

- In a small bowl, whisk together olive oil, lemon juice, Dijon mustard, salt, and pepper to make the dressing.

- Flake the cooked salmon and add it to the salad.

- Drizzle the lemon Dijon dressing over the salad and toss to combine. Serve immediately.

Spaghetti Squash Carbonara

Ingredients:

- 1 large spaghetti squash

- 4 slices bacon, diced

- 2 cloves garlic, minced

- 2 eggs

- 1/2 cup grated Parmesan cheese

- 1/4 cup chopped fresh parsley

- Salt and pepper to taste

Instructions:

- Preheat the oven to 400°F (200°C). Cut the spaghetti squash in half lengthwise and remove the seeds.

- Place the squash halves, cut side down, on a baking sheet. Bake for 30-40 minutes or until tender.

- While the squash is baking, cook the diced bacon in a skillet over medium heat until crispy. Add minced garlic and cook for an additional minute. Remove from heat.

- In a bowl, whisk together eggs, grated Parmesan cheese, chopped parsley, salt, and pepper.

- Scrape the cooked spaghetti squash with a fork to create "noodles". Add the spaghetti squash noodles to the skillet with the bacon and garlic.

- Pour the egg mixture over the spaghetti squash and toss until well combined. The heat from the squash will cook the eggs and create a creamy sauce.

- Serve spaghetti squash carbonara immediately, garnished with additional Parmesan cheese and parsley if desired.

Tuna and White Bean Salad

Ingredients:

- 2 cans (5 oz each) tuna, drained

- 1 can (15 oz) cannellini beans, drained and rinsed

- 1 red bell pepper, diced

- 1/4 cup red onion, finely chopped

- 2 tablespoons chopped fresh parsley

- 2 tablespoons olive oil

- 1 tablespoon lemon juice

- 1 teaspoon Dijon mustard

- Salt and pepper to taste

Instructions:

- In a large bowl, combine drained tuna, cannellini beans, diced red bell pepper, chopped red onion, and chopped parsley.

- In a small bowl, whisk together olive oil, lemon juice, Dijon mustard, salt, and pepper to make the dressing.

- Pour the dressing over the tuna and white bean mixture and toss to combine.

- Serve tuna and white bean salad chilled or at room temperature.

Mediterranean Stuffed Zucchini

Ingredients:

- 4 medium zucchini

- 1 can (15 oz) chickpeas, drained and rinsed

- 1 cup cherry tomatoes, halved

- 1/4 cup sliced black olives

- 1/4 cup crumbled feta cheese

- 2 tablespoons chopped fresh parsley

- 2 tablespoons olive oil

- 1 tablespoon lemon juice

- 1 teaspoon dried oregano

- Salt and pepper to taste

Instructions:

- Preheat the oven to 375°F (190°C). Cut each zucchini in half lengthwise and scoop out the seeds to create a hollow center.

- In a bowl, combine drained chickpeas, halved cherry tomatoes, sliced black olives, crumbled feta cheese, chopped parsley, olive oil, lemon juice, dried oregano, salt, and pepper.

- Fill each hollowed-out zucchini half with the chickpea mixture.

- Place stuffed zucchini halves on a baking sheet lined with parchment paper. Bake for 20-25 minutes or until zucchini is tender.

- Serve Mediterranean stuffed zucchini hot, garnished with additional chopped parsley if desired.

Lemon Herb Roasted Chicken Thighs

Ingredients:

- 6 chicken thighs, bone-in and skin-on

- Zest of 1 lemon

- Juice of 1 lemon

- 2 cloves garlic, minced

- 2 tablespoons chopped fresh rosemary

- 2 tablespoons chopped fresh thyme

- 2 tablespoons olive oil

- Salt and pepper to taste

Instructions:

- Preheat the oven to 400°F (200°C). Line a baking sheet with parchment paper.

- In a bowl, whisk together lemon zest, lemon juice, minced garlic, chopped rosemary, chopped thyme, olive oil, salt, and pepper.

- Place chicken thighs on the prepared baking sheet. Brush the lemon herb mixture over the chicken thighs.

- Roast in the oven for 25-30 minutes or until the chicken is golden brown and cooked through.

- Serve lemon herb roasted chicken thighs hot.

Chia Seed Pudding with Berries

Ingredients:

- 1/4 cup chia seeds

- 1 cup unsweetened almond milk

- 1 tablespoon maple syrup or honey

- 1/2 teaspoon vanilla extract

- Mixed berries for topping (such as strawberries, blueberries, and raspberries)

Instructions:

- In a bowl, mix chia seeds, almond milk, maple syrup (or honey), and vanilla extract until well combined.

- Cover and refrigerate for at least 2 hours or overnight, stirring occasionally to prevent clumping.

- Once the chia pudding has thickened to your desired consistency, divide it into serving bowls or jars.

- Top with mixed berries before serving. Enjoy chilled!

Sesame Ginger Turkey Lettuce Wraps

Ingredients:

- 1 lb ground turkey

- 2 tablespoons soy sauce

- 1 tablespoon sesame oil

- 2 cloves garlic, minced

- 1 tablespoon grated ginger

- 1 cup mixed vegetables (such as bell peppers, water chestnuts, and carrots), diced

- Butter lettuce leaves, for wrapping

- Sliced green onions for garnish

- Sesame seeds for garnish

Instructions:

- In a skillet, heat sesame oil over medium heat. Add minced garlic and grated ginger, and cook until fragrant.

- Add ground turkey to the skillet and cook until browned, breaking it apart with a spoon.

- Stir in diced mixed vegetables and soy sauce. Cook for an additional 3-5 minutes until the vegetables are tender.

- Spoon the turkey mixture onto butter lettuce leaves. Garnish with sliced green onions and sesame seeds before serving.

Asian-Inspired Cucumber Salad

Ingredients:

- 2 cucumbers, thinly sliced
- 1/4 cup rice vinegar
- 1 tablespoon soy sauce
- 1 teaspoon sesame oil
- 1 teaspoon honey
- 1/2 teaspoon grated ginger
- 1 clove garlic, minced
- 1 tablespoon sesame seeds
- Sliced green onions for garnish

Instructions:

- In a large bowl, whisk together rice vinegar, soy sauce, sesame oil, honey, grated ginger, and minced garlic to make the dressing.

- Add thinly sliced cucumbers to the bowl and toss until evenly coated with the dressing.

- Sprinkle sesame seeds over the cucumber salad and toss again to combine.

- Garnish with sliced green onions before serving.

Creamy Garlic Mushroom Risotto

Ingredients:

- 1 cup Arborio rice

- 4 cups vegetable broth

- 2 tablespoons olive oil

- 2 tablespoons butter

- 2 cloves garlic, minced

- 8 oz mushrooms, sliced

- 1/4 cup grated Parmesan cheese

- 2 tablespoons chopped fresh parsley

- Salt and pepper to taste

Instructions:

- In a saucepan, heat vegetable broth over medium heat and keep it warm.

- In a separate large skillet, heat olive oil and butter over medium heat. Add minced garlic and sliced mushrooms. Cook until mushrooms are golden brown.

- Add Arborio rice to the skillet and cook, stirring frequently, for 1-2 minutes.

- Ladle warm vegetable broth into the skillet, one ladleful at a time, stirring constantly until absorbed before adding more. Continue this process until the rice is creamy and tender, about 20-25 minutes.

- Stir in grated Parmesan cheese and chopped parsley. Season with salt and pepper to taste.

- Serve creamy garlic mushroom risotto hot.

Miso Glazed Tofu with Stir-Fried Vegetables

Ingredients:

- 1 block firm tofu, drained and pressed, cut into cubes

- 2 tablespoons miso paste

- 2 tablespoons soy sauce

- 1 tablespoon maple syrup

- 1 tablespoon rice vinegar

- 1 tablespoon sesame oil

- 2 cloves garlic, minced

- 1 tablespoon grated ginger

- Assorted vegetables (such as bell peppers, broccoli, and snap peas), sliced

- Cooked brown rice for serving

Instructions:

- In a bowl, whisk together miso paste, soy sauce, maple syrup, rice vinegar, sesame oil, minced garlic, and grated ginger.

- Marinate tofu cubes in the miso mixture for at least 30 minutes.

- Heat a skillet over medium-high heat and add marinated tofu cubes. Cook until browned and crispy on all sides.

- In the same skillet, stir-fry assorted vegetables until tender-crisp.

- Serve miso glazed tofu over cooked brown rice with stir-fried vegetables.

Barley and Mushroom Soup

Ingredients:

- 1 cup pearl barley, rinsed

- 8 cups vegetable broth

- 2 tablespoons olive oil

- 1 onion, diced

- 2 carrots, diced

- 2 celery stalks, diced

- 8 oz mushrooms, sliced

- 2 cloves garlic, minced

- 1 teaspoon dried thyme

- Salt and pepper to taste

- Chopped fresh parsley for garnish

Instructions:

- In a large pot, heat olive oil over medium heat. Add diced onion, carrots, and celery. Cook until softened.

- Add sliced mushrooms and minced garlic to the pot. Cook until mushrooms are tender.

- Stir in pearl barley and dried thyme. Cook for 1-2 minutes.

- Pour in vegetable broth and bring to a boil. Reduce heat and simmer for about 45-50 minutes or until barley is tender.

- Season with salt and pepper to taste.

- Serve barley and mushroom soup hot, garnished with chopped fresh parsley.

Cajun Shrimp and Vegetable Skewers

Ingredients:

- 1 lb large shrimp, peeled and deveined

- 2 bell peppers (assorted colors), cut into chunks

- 1 red onion, cut into chunks

- 1 zucchini, sliced

- 2 tablespoons olive oil

- 1 tablespoon Cajun seasoning

- Salt and pepper to taste

Instructions:

- Preheat grill to medium-high heat.

- In a bowl, toss shrimp, bell peppers, red onion, and zucchini with olive oil and Cajun seasoning until evenly coated.

- Thread shrimp, bell peppers, red onion, and zucchini onto skewers.

- Season skewers with salt and pepper.

- Grill skewers for 2-3 minutes per side, or until shrimp are

  cooked through and vegetables are tender.

- Serve Cajun shrimp and vegetable skewers hot.

THANKS   FOR

READING

THIS BOOK.

www.ingramcontent.com/pod-product-compliance
Lightning Source LLC
Chambersburg PA
CBHW050826250726
48653CB00006B/2458